MEN'S HEALTH

Nester Murira

1

This book will answer many questions men may have about their health.

Table of Contents

Chapter 12

Your Food and Health

Chapter 1

BECOMING A MAN

Adulthood is a process that starts at puberty. Ideally this process should be a guided process in which adult males induct a young man into adulthood through informed discussion and mentoring as well as through observation. However in some families, young men may grow and become men without this much needed guidance on socially accepted behaviors, language and character.

Some young men may depend on instinct to express themselves while others may learn male behaviors from friends. It is important that a young man is guided into manhood by a mentor who could be the father or an older brother or a guardian. It is therefore important that mature men understand the changes that occur in the transitional period from puberty to manhood. This knowledge helps in explaining and answering questions from young people. It is important that fathers have a good relationship with their sons so that they can discuss freely about any subject of adulthood. It is best that a child learns facts of life from a parent, a close relative or guided lessons in churches, youth clubs and colleges than from friends.

Physical Changes in Boys at Puberty

Puberty is the stage of transition from childhood to adulthood. It is marked by a rapid physical growth and secondary development of all organs in the body including sexual organs. This phase of development is influenced by the Growth Hormone or Somatotrophic Hormone and the sex hormones, Gonadotrophic Hormones. Both the Somatotrophic and Gonadotrophic hormones are produced by the anterior lobe of the master gland or the pituitary gland that sits at the base of the skull. These hormones are produced in increasing amounts from the age of eight years, to influence body development.

The hormones bring about significant changes transforming a young boy into a young adult. This growth spurt may bring about a mixture of confusion and excitement in a young person as a young man becomes aware of the physical changes in his body. There are changes in all parts of the body and in all the systems of the body.

- The genital organs are directly influenced by the sex hormones and increase in size. The male reproductive system becomes fully developed.
- There is maturation and enlargement of the testes which descend down from the abdomen through a small opening in the groin, the inguinal canal to

the scrotum below the groins where they should remain for the rest of the male adult's life.

- Sometimes testes remain in the abdomen, an abnormal situation called undescended testes. This is corrected through by doctors through surgery. If the condition is not corrected early, one may have infertility. It is important that at puberty young men feel the testes in the scrotum and report to health personnel if the scrotal sac remains empty when all the other signs of puberty are present.

- The testes function efficiently with low temperatures. The temperature of the scrotal sac is much lower than the rest of the body to enable production and maturation of spermatozoa or the male seed. It is advisable that young men avoid tight underwear that generates heat and alters scrotal temperature and opt for loose airy clothes. Excessive heat to the genital organs alters sperm production and viability. It is necessary that young people who work in furnaces and long distance drivers of haulages take time to enjoy free fresh air and cool their body temperatures.

- The inguinal opening should close as the young man grows. If the inguinal canal fails to close tightly it may be a cause for inguinal hernias, in which a small loop of the bowel slips down out of the abdominal wall and appears as a swelling in the groin. The swelling can be temporary and may disappear when one lies flat on the back and swells once more when one coughs or lifts something heavy. Inguinal hernias are common in weight lifters and athletes. Occasionally a loop of the bowel can slip down as far as the scrotal sac where it is seen as a sudden painful swelling. The scrotal sac on one side looks abnormally larger than the other. This is an emergency and one must seek health services without delay. All hernias are corrected by surgery.

- The cords that suspend the testes (man's balls), can sometimes twist (torsion) causing extreme scrotal or groin pain. Torsion becomes an emergency requiring immediate surgery to release the knot.

- At puberty, the Follicle Stimulating hormone from the anterior lobe of the pituitary gland stimulates the seminiferous tubules in the testes to become active and fully functional glands that produce the male reproductive seed, the *spermatozoa*.

- Spermatozoa swim in a white fluid, *semen*, which is produced by seminal ducts in the testes and by the prostate gland.

- A second male sex hormone, The Interstitial Cell Stimulating hormone is produced by the anterior lobe of the pituitary gland and stimulates testicular tissue (the little balls in the scrotum), to produce the male sex hormone, testosterone.

Functions of Testosterone

- **Testosterone is responsible for the marked developmental changes in a young man (the maleness) development of internal male sexual organs, male characteristics, and male sexual behaviors. Boys will begin to grow a little hair on the chin which will later become beard. Hair also grows in armpits and on the pubic area.**

- **Testosterone influences the male metabolism especially protein digestion and use in the body**
  and together with the Growth hormone influence muscular development in the young man especially the typical broad

shoulders and the strong male muscles. Boys appetite generally increases and the strong thigh muscles.

- Testosterone is responsible for sexual desire, the need to attract and be noticed by the opposite sex and the drive to physically engage in sexual activity.

- Boys dream of erotic scenes and discharge semen with spermatozoa in their sleep, commonly referred to as wet dreams. Should a young man have sexual intercourse from this stage of development and onwards, he is capable of becoming a father. Boys have a tendency to have a crush over older women at this stage.

- The young man's voice deepens, a development commonly known as 'breaking of voice' and the voice box or Adam's apple becomes visibly enlarged.

- There is an observable increase in height caused by the combined effect of the growth hormone on long bones and the effect of the male hormone testosterone

- Testosterone plays a part in fluid and salts (electrolyte) balance in the kidneys.

- Young men are known to have more difficulty adjusting to the sudden influx of the hormones at puberty than girls do.

- Testosterone triggers the urge to experiment with the developed organs, hence the need for adolescent sexual health education around puberty for both young men and women.

Questions and Beliefs

There are untrue and uninformed beliefs and myths that circulate in societies that may mislead you as a young person in your quest to understand sexuality. It is important that as a young person you seek answers to the questions and anxieties you may have about sexuality from informed sources such as health personnel.

How can I prove that my sperms are viable and that I am fertile?

A healthy young person who has had healthy secondary sexual development and has not experienced infections of the genital system should not have undue fears about fertility neither should he need to prove anything about fertility to anyone. These anxieties should not put pressure on young people to find an excuse for indulging in unplanned, illicit and wanton sexual behaviors. Proof of fertility will be seen when one is ready to start a family. Should one have a problem then, health personnel will conduct the necessary investigations and provide relevant advice and remedy where possible.

Is the appearance of one's semen suggestive of one's fertility status?

The semen is fluid which provides a medium and transport of the male seed from the testicles through the male reproductive system. One cannot see the male seed with the naked eye; sperms can only be seen under a microscope. The semen can therefore not provide one with answers about fertility. Tests on fertility are done in adults after a doctor's advice and the specific couple's consent.

What if one produces small amounts of semen; is this cause for concern? One may produce any amount of semen but what is important is the health of the actual seed contained in the semen which can only be seen in laboratories by specialists using special equipment.

Men and Virginity

In some societies, there is a fuss about girls being virgins at marriage but there is no insistence that a young man be a virgin too. Virginity is important in both partners as it increases trust between partners and reduces the incidence of sexually transmitted diseases including HIV and AIDS in married couples. It is not cool to have many girlfriends as this is a sure recipe for contracting sexually transmitted diseases.

If a young man can have several girlfriends before marriage, and father several children out of wedlock, he cannot be trusted to be a faithful husband to his wife. It is the responsibility of mature men and fathers to advise young men to respect their bodies and be faithful partners to their spouses.

Chapter 2

MEN'S RESPONSIBILITIES IN SEXUAL AND REPRODUCTIVE HEALTH

Sexual Responsibility

Responsible sexual behavior is having knowledge about one's sexual organs and how they function, understanding the consequences of sexual activity, planning for sexual activity by taking precautions of negative consequences such as unwanted unplanned pregnancies, sexually transmitted diseases, accepting the responsibilities that come with sexual activity and only engaging in sexual activity after considering and accepting the responsibilities.

Understanding your partner

A man needs to understand women's sexual and reproductive health in order to understand his partner's response to sexual issues.

Men can be excited and stimulated by visual excitement of the woman, her clothing, gait, facial and body looks while women may get excited when they see a man they fancy but may not be as spontaneous as men and may need to think about sex. The sexual response in women can be described as having four phases. These are: *excitement, plateau, orgasm and resolution*.

- Women get excited and warm up to the sexual act through touch and foreplay.

This stage is important to make the woman's system ready, get her muscles relaxed and her genital lubricants flow to enable smooth painless and enjoyable sexual act. It is possible for men to get carried away and rush into a sexual act before the partner is ready. The writer has spoken to many frustrated women whose partners rush to conclude the sexual act while the woman is still warming up. This causes sexual dissatisfaction and discord in a relationship.

- *Orgasm or the climax* in the pleasure is the same in men and women except that men ejaculate semen while women's organs go into a spasm as the woman reaches the height of sexual pleasure.

The excitement is brought about by nerve impulses from the lumbar region of the back contracting the pelvic muscles rhythmically.

- The phase of resolution or relaxation follows successful ejaculation and orgasm.

Sexual needs

Women have the same sexual needs as men but women may conceal their feelings because that may be the expected norm in their culture or society or because they are shy.

- It is desirable that partners are open with each other about sexual expectations and know what they want from a sexual relationship. Free discussion about sexual activity is encouraged between partners so that they understand each other's sexual needs and what is right for them.

- Psychological, social and cultural influences may determine some people's sexual behaviours and sexual drive. Women are more influenced by psychosocial factors in their sexual behavior than men.

- In some cultures women are made to believe that in a relationship, the man's demands are more important than theirs, that a man is the expert and that they should submit to their partner's sexual demands as a rule. In some cultures, women may be manipulated for the man's pleasure and are expected to be the passive partner who is less demanding and wait for the man to initiate for a sexual act. There should be free expression of the desire to have sexual intercourse from both partners.

- Men should consider the needs of their partners as many women confess that men are aggressive sexually and worry more about displaying their sexual prowess. More often men may get carried away with their desires and may forget or show little concern about the feelings of the woman, her pleasure or satisfaction.

- There are many women who never realize orgasm or pleasure in a sexual act because the man is in a hurry; there is no foreplay or communication about each other's sexual needs

Sexual Problems

While most adults are full of energy and keen on sexual activity, there are however, exceptions to the usual behavior where there are sexual problems. It is not every young couple that is open to discuss sexual problems when they arise. It is however important that couples are aware of likely sexual problems so that they can seek help. The only way to access help is to talk about the prevailing problem. Couples can access help from health personnel should they have sexual health problems. Health personnel can only assist their clients in sexual issues if their clients freely express their sexual problems.

Dysfunction of arousal and Orgasm in your partner

The human sexual response is influenced by previous experiences, memories, emotions, associations and thoughts and in females, the phase of the female cycle. Women may feel disinterested in sex during the early days of the female cycle which is influenced by the hormone oestrogen. The female hormone oestrogen, produced in the first half of the female cycle causes in the female system, muscle tension, low sexual desire (libido) and failure to reach orgasm.

- Women on combined pill may experience tension headaches, poor relaxation and poor arousal. Causes of sexual dysfunction in the female may therefore be due to disinterest in sexual activity due to low levels of the female hormone, progesterone at this time of the cycle.

- Towards the middle of the cycle as more progesterone is produced, women in general experience a gradual increase in desire for sexual activity.

- Many women respond well to prolonged foreplay and may reach orgasm. Women are generally more relaxed, receptive to sexual arousal and enjoy sexual intercourse during the second phase of the female cycle influenced by the hormone progesterone.

- Where adequate precautions to prevent pregnancy have not been taken, the fear of falling pregnant may cause tension and poor arousal.
- Ignorance by either partner of genital anatomy, functions, technique of arousal and stimulation, inability and lack of experience to achieve sexual satisfaction play a major role in arousal problems.
- There are other factors that may cause a woman to be tensed up such as having feelings of inadequacy, fear of loss of control and religious inhibitions, marital discord, anger, guilt, depression, stressful situations such as impending

divorce, or stress due to the death of a loved one.

- Secondary causes of arousal dysfunction in a woman could arise from anxiety about performance or ability to please partner. Interpersonal causes such as failure to communicate effectively with the partner about desired foreplay, desired sexual positions and the length of the sexual act may cause sexual tension and failure to relax and reach orgasm.

- Tension due to physical causes such as localized infections that cause swelling or inflammation of parts of the female organs like swelling inside the uterus,(endometriosis), Swelling of the bladder (cystitis), pelvic inflammatory diseases, swelling of the vaginal walls (vaginitis)may cause poor arousal.

- Diseases such as hypothyroidism (low levels of the hormone thyroxine), diabetes, and nervous disorders are known to depress sexual drive in women.

- Drugs such as oral contraceptives especially the combined pill suppresses sexual desire, drugs that treat hypertension and tranquilizers cause muscle relaxation and suppress sexual desire.

- Surgery on female organs may bring about a feeling of inadequacy in women e.g. removal of the female tubes (salpingectomy), removal of the ovaries(oophrectomy), removal of the breast (mastectomy), and removal of the uterus, (hysterectomy).

- Poor arousal may be due to dislike of partner, caused by poor sexual technique, bad smell from mouth, alcohol, sweat.

- Failed orgasm especially in women is common especially where there is poor communication and the man is driven by his desire to ejaculate before the partner is properly stimulated and close to orgasm.

- A couple can seek help for arousal problems, and must inform health personnel about detailed history of the pattern of one's menstrual cycle, one's contraceptive method and a detailed sexual history revealing one's sexual beliefs, myths and expectations from the partner to assist in identifying the problem.

- A physical examination will be done as part of the search for the problem and reaching for a solution. An open discussion may be all that is required and this should be possible without need to see health personnel.

- Should the problem persist, a woman should expect to have hormonal levels tests especially where the history and physical examination results are suggestive of inadequate hormonal flow.

- The doctor will always explain the findings and should involve you as a couple in discussion that enables you to make an informed decision about management of the condition.

- Sexual activity is encouraged between trusted partners who are ready and agreed to the activity.

- Satisfactory sexual activity ideally cements relationships, prevent marital discord, and prevent extramarital sexual relationships and polygamy. Patterns of sexual behaviour and norms may be influenced by the culture of a given society and the environment.

Sexual Precautions

- Sexual activity has consequences that one has to be prepared for such as pregnancy, wanted or unwanted unplanned pregnancy and sexually transmitted disease including HIV.

- There are several methods of contraception available for both men and women to prevent unwanted pregnancy or delay pregnancy until one is ready for it.

- There are methods of contraception that also prevent sexually transmitted diseases.

- If you feel that you are ready for sexual activity, take precautions to prevent unwanted unpleasant and serious consequences of irresponsible sexual behaviour.

There is no reason why your partner should fall pregnant if she does not want to. It is equally the man's responsibility to prevent pregnancy as much as it is a woman's.

The Condom

The condom or sheath, or rubber tube is the only method that prevents pregnancy and sexually transmitted infections at the same time.

It is the best method for young people who do not wish to start taking hormones early in life.

- The condom is a method that does not need a prescription or measurement of one's body structures.
- The condom is readily available in shops, chemists, hospitals, GP's, health centres.

- The condom is the best method when a couple wishes to prevent or delay pregnancy.
- The condom is easily the best method to use while one's partner recovers from a pregnancy as one does not need to see health personnel to start using it.
- The condom can also be used when your partner is starting on a hormone method for the first two weeks to allow the hormone blood levels to reach safe levels that prevent pregnancy.
- The condom should be used to prevent contracting sexually transmitted diseases.

How to use the male condom

- The man must wear the condom when aroused and before the sexual act. Your partner can help you apply it as part of foreplay.
- There is no need for use of oil or jel, the condom is well lubricated.
- One size fits all, there is no need to get measured for size
- It is important to hold the top of the condom as you ease out of your partner to prevent spillage of semen onto your partner's organs.
- It is important to wrap the condom in tissue paper and flush it in the toilet or dispose of it in the rubbish bin.

- A condom should be used once for one act and disposed of. It <u>should not</u> be washed or used repeatedly.
- Unused condoms must be stored away from heat and the sun. Rubber is weakened and destroyed by heat.
- There is no reason why a man should contract sexually transmitted diseases because the condom is available everywhere.

Female condom

There is a condom for women too.

The female condom prevents both pregnancy and sexually transmitted infections.

- The female condom must be worn before the sexual act.

- There are other methods like the foams and pessaries that a young woman can introduce inside her female genital organ before sexual intercourse.
- The foam and pessary must be repeated should there be need to have another sexual act.
- Women have many other alternative reliable choices of methods of contraception that they can use.
- It is important to check with one's partner that she is protected from an unwanted pregnancy before a sexual act.
- There is no reason why one's sexual partner should fall pregnant if the necessary precautions are taken.

Vasectomy (The Snip)

- Vasectomy is an effective family planning method in which the man decides to take responsibility to plan his family when he and his partner decide that their family is complete and the man does not wish to father any more babies.

- Vasectomy is a minor surgical operation done in men who do not wish to continue to father babies.

What is involved in the operation?

- The operation (snip) takes a few minutes and one can go home immediately. The tube , (Vas deferens) extends from the male seed basket (testes), one from each testis and carries the male seed over the bladder and down the posterior part of the bladder to open into the urethra below the bladder.

- The two tiny tubes, the vas deferens, one from each testis, are snipped or cut using a surgical blade just behind the scrotum, and tied using suturing material so that the male seed passage is blocked.

- One has to give this procedure a good thought before making an informed decision to have the operation because this procedure is permanent or irreversible, meaning that one can no longer father babies thereafter.

When can one start having sexual relationships following this procedure?

- Vasectomy is a minor procedure and one can have normal sexual relationships as soon as one has no pain, usually within seven days, but, one must use a condom for at least three weeks to ensure that one's system is completely free of the male seed.

Can one still enjoy sexual relationships after the operation?

There is nothing to stop one from enjoying sexual relationship after the operation after all one's mind is at peace knowing that the activity will not result in a pregnancy.

Can one ejaculate semen after the operation?

- In normal life, a small amount of semen is produced by the testes to allow for the male seed to swim through the vas deferens. The large amount of semen is produced outside the testes by the seminal vesicles and the prostate gland below the bladder.

- Semen will continue to be produced as usual and is ejaculated during the sexual act.

- After vasectomy semen will be just a fluid without the male seed.

What happens to the male seed after vasectomy?

The seed is re-absorbed and destroyed in the testes. This does not affect the size of the testes or change them in any way or cause any disease or pain at all.

Does one feel different or feel a lesser man after vasectomy?

One feels as normal as usual. There is no need for one to feel a lesser man or feeling low. The only change in the person is that they can no longer father babies. This is a couple's secret and decision and should not cause any worries.

Sexual Abuse

Sexual abuse includes touching, fondling, patting, of an individual's body, contact with one's sexual organs either by touching or penetration or forcing oneself on an individual or illicit sexual assault without consent.

- Anyone including trusted members of families, members of society entrusted with the care of children in schools, and refugee camps as well as social deviants and perverts have been reported to sexually abuse young people.
- There is no need for men to behave in such animal like sexual behaviour. Real men, ask mature girls for a sexual relationship. Real men control their sexual desires and do not take advantage of innocent helpless children or girls. Sex is for adults who both know the consequences of their behavior.

- Sexually abusing children is punishable by law. Men could control their sexual desire and avoid hurting little girls.

Incest

Incestuous relationships are sexual relationship between related people or close family members.

- Even if yours is a broken homes, a girl child should not be taken advantage of by a parent, some guardians, brothers and uncles entrusted with the welfare of the child. There are more women that men in the world. Any man who wants a mature sexual partner can get one. Let children be children. Respect a relative. Don't behave like an animal which knows no boundaries. Don't force yourself on a relative, it makes you a pervert, undesirable in society and a sex offender.

- Some misguided family members believe incestuous relationships bring luck in business, in misfortune, and in illness. Sexual abuse of a relative does not bring any luck or relieve any illness; neither does it solve anyone's problems.

- Sexual abuse robs a young person of her innocence; it confuses the young person and may cause emotional instability.

- The young girl can be exposed to sexually transmitted diseases including the deadly HIV/AIDS.

Rape

- Rape is forced sexual act without the consent of one partner. It is an offence and punishable by law.
- One should be able to freely choose their sexual partner.
- Sexual activity is more enjoyable if you get consent from a mature person. Respect other people. Women have a right to have sexual intercourse with a man of their choice.
- Decent enjoyable sexual intercourse is every person's right and that right must not be taken away by some misguided man. Rape does not make a man macho or desirable or respected. It makes a man a social deviant, a social outcast and undesirable.

- Any female wants to be respected and her rights respected. Men can control their desires for sex until they get a mature person who is willing to be their sexual partner.
- Men must learn to make themselves presentable, attractive and eligible so that they can be accepted by women when they approach them.

Sex Slaves

- There are perverts the world over who abduct young girls and keep them in secluded places for the perverts' sexual needs.
- Take interest in who your daughter communicates with on internet and what the subject of the communication is.

Young girls can be lured by sexual perverts pretending to be their age mates and abducted through internet communication.

- It is important to know your daughter's friends and their parents. It cannot be overstated that young girls need close parental protection.

- It is safest to take your young girl to school and leave her in the school yard and make it your responsibility to collect her from school.

- When you go shopping or for an outing with your daughter, keep your daughter within sight.

- When you are going away, ensure that you leave your daughter with people you know and trust.

Early marriages

Early marriages are usually arranged marriages of elderly men and children before the age of sixteen. Early marriages occur in some cultures where girls in particular are married off to elderly men before full developmental potential due to cultural practices, as a price to pay off debts, in exchange for food in famine hit societies, and to avenge angry spirits of the wronged dead in some tribes.

- It is up to parents to protect young girls from early marriages. Parents and especially fathers should resist the practice and refuse to allow their daughters into such arrangements at any age in a child's life.

- It is a young girl's right to choose a life partner of her choice when she is ready to do that.
- Marriage before a young girl turns twenty is early teenage marriage. It is not advisable as one's body has not yet reached its full growth potential, besides, the young person is likely to be exposed to many complications related to sexual and reproductive health such as sexually transmitted diseases including HIV, and loss of life.

Cultural practices

There are some cultural inheritance practices which may predispose young girls to sexual abuse and sexually transmitted diseases including HIV/AIDS.

- Some cultures and religious sects persuade young girls into taking over a sister's husband or an aunt's husband after the death of a relative, or push young girls into a polygamous relationship. This is sexual abuse; it exposes a young girl to sexually transmitted infections including HIV.

- It is also sexual abuse for a young man to be expected to take over an older brother's wife in the event of a brother dying and leaving a wife behind. This exposes one to sexually transmitted infections including HIV.

- There are dangers of forcing a young girl to be married off to old men in the society for whatever reason, economic, religious or cultural. It is everyone's responsibility, fathers included to oppose such tradition that disadvantages young girls.

- Forcing a person into a sexual act is an offense. Marrying off young girls to older men or forcing a young person into such a relationship is a crime which must be reported to police and other human rights organizations because it is sexual and mental abuse.

Beliefs

Some societies may believe in practices that make young girls vulnerable. Parents should be on the lookout for any beliefs and practices that expose their

daughters to sexual abuse and condemn
them in the strongest terms.

Chapter3

MALE FERTILITY

A person is considered infertile after living together with a spouse continuously for two years having regular normal sexual relationships at the right time of the female cycle.

- Women are highly fertile from around the fourteenth day after a monthly period. The female egg is released from the female egg basket (ovulation) around the fourteenth day after a period. The egg is in the female's genital system for at least seven days. This is the best time to try to achieve a pregnancy.

- The timing of these days is very important as one may think they are infertile when they are trying for pregnancy at the wrong time.

What is male fertility?

Male fertility is determined by ability to produce adequate numbers of male seed (spermatozoa).

- It is estimated that normal sperm count should be over 50 million sperms per millilitre of semen. Figures below this count may result in male sterility.
- The male seed must have a normal size, a normal shape and must be able to swim to meet the female egg and fertilize it.
- Only one sperm(male seed) fertilizes the egg but sperm are required in large numbers to produce a substance that

makes the egg soft to enable one sperm to fertilize the egg.

What may cause one to produce a small amount of sperms?

Inadequate hormones.

- Men may have problems in producing adequate amounts of testicular stimulating hormone from the pituitary gland to stimulate testicular cells to produce the male hormone testosterone that is essential in the production of the male seed and maturation of the male seed.
- The male seed may be deformed and weak and fails to reach the female egg to fertilize it.

- The male tubes male be blocked by previous infection and the male seed fails to reach the woman.

- The testes need adequate amounts of Follicle Stimulating Hormone from the lower part of the brain (Pituitary gland) to produce sperms.

- Inadequate stimulation of the testes by the hormone result in low production of sperms. The second hormone from the pituitary gland (ICSH) Intersticial Cell Stimulating Hormone causes production of the male hormone testosterone by the testes.

- Testosterone causes the male seed to mature. In the absence of adequate amounts of testosterone, sperms are fragile and may not have a normal shape, size and ability to swim vigorously.

Blockage in the testes

Sexually transmitted infections may leave testes swollen or blocked by pus and when healing occurs, the testicular tissues stick together, form scars and block the flow of sperms making the individual sterile or infertile.

- It is important that one avoids sexually transmitted diseases through having one faithful sexual partner, or using a condom.
- Should one partner contract a sexually transmitted infection, it is imperative that both partners are treated thoroughly until the infection clears.

How can one tell that he is infertile?

- Both partners have to have tests by health specialists who can examine the man and collect specimens to check the amounts of hormones being produced by one's body, do a sperm count and examine one's organs for normalcy.

- Using one's eyes to examine the colour or thickness of one's semen will not tell you whether you are fertile or not.

- Special tests must be done and specimens examined by powerful machines in laboratories to determine poor hormonal function and low sperm counts.

- One's partner is also thoroughly examined and tested.

Discharge of semen does not mean that a man is fertile.

- Semen is a fluid that transports the male seed.
- Semen may not contain the male seed if the testes fail to produce the seed.
- Some semen is produced by testicular tissue and most of it is produced by the prostate gland.

You and your partner must be examined by health personnel and must go through suggested tests to find the cause of infertility.

It is important to access information on the male reproductive system as well as the female cycle and time   sexual activity at the advised period of the month the female is most fertile..

- It is important that a couple lives together continuously while trying for a pregnancy.
- Several investigations of both male and female reproductive systems are done to exclude infections, blockages and tumours of the genital organs.
- Investigations on the flow of hormones,(hormonal assays), are done. Supplementary hormones can be given to any of the partners who may not be producing adequate amounts of hormones.
- The man's semen is examined to see the amounts and structure of the sperms to ascertain if they are healthy.

- The female system is examined. It is important to ascertain if the flow of the female hormones is adequate to enable the ovaries to ovulate.

- Assisted fertility can be discussed between the couple and an obstetrician to enable a couple to achieve a pregnancy.

Please note that the sex of the baby is determined by the male seed and not the female. It is the man who bears the 'Y' gene that makes male babies.

After these tests, can one father a child?

- Low hormonal flow can be stimulated by supplements prescribed by health specialists. Blockage of any part of the testes cannot be reversed. There are alternatives to become a father through artificial methods.

- Details of artificial methods of achieving fatherhood can be discussed with the health specialists.

Chapter 4

SEXUALLY TRANSMITTED INFECTIONS (STIS)

Sexually transmitted infections are diseases spread from one person to another through sexual contact. The most common causes of infection are:

Bacteria, Viruses, Fungus Protozoa

Chlamydia Infection

This infection is now the most common of all bacterial STIs.

- Many people with Chlamydial infection, however, have few or no symptoms of infection.

- Chlamydial infection causes an abnormal watery and itchy genital discharge
- One feels a burning sensation on passing urine.
- If untreated Chlamydial infection may lead to pelvic inflammatory disease (PID), that causes aches and pains and swelling in the internal female organs.
- One experiences pain during intercourse (dyspareunia.
- The female tubes are most affected, become swollen and may collect pus inside them causing blockage of tubes.
- As the tubes heal, scar tissue that prevents the normal function of the tube forms and further narrows.

- Blocked and narrowed tubes are the most common causes of ectopic pregnancy and infertility in women).
- In men Chlamydia infection causes swelling of testes, orchitis which interferes with production of spermatozoa and may cause low sperm production, a cause of male infertility.

Genital Herpes

Genital herpes is caused by herpes simplex virus (HSV).

- The infected person may feel a r burning sensation in the groins, buttocks, and genital region.
- The groin lymph nodes are swollen.
- One experiences a rise in temperature and chills.

- <u>Painful blisters</u> appear on the genital organs in clusters.
- The blisters open to become painful weepy sores. The sores may become infected and look dirty with patches of pus. The sores can be washed and painted with antiseptics.
- The herpes sores usually disappear within two to three weeks.
- The virus remains in the body for life and the blisters and sores may recur from time to time.
- Suppressive Antiviral therapy can be used to prevent re-occurrences but these do not destroy the virus.
- Both partners must be treated
- Genital herpes can be transmitted to newborn babies during childbirth.

- Untreated HSV infection in newborns can result in mental retardation and death.

Syphilis

Syphilis is a curable sexually transmitted infection caused by the bacteria

- Early symptoms of syphilis may go undetected because they are very mild and disappear spontaneously.
- The major symptom is usually <u>a painless open sore</u> with raised margins that appears on soft tissue such as the penis, the vagina, lips, gums, under the nails and around the anus.
- A rash that covers the whole body including the face and neck appears.

- The various internal organs such as the heart are also affected causing syphilitic heart disease.

- The brain and central nervous system are affected resulting in paralysis of limbs and mental disturbances.

- Large open wounds especially on the legs appear due to poor blood flow and poor nerve sensation.

- In young women syphilis is a major cause of abortions, stillbirth and death of the newborn babies.

- Babies born with syphilis may have a rash all over the body. The babies usually have abnormal features of the internal organs, and especially facial bones. The newborn have difficulty in breathing (snuffles).

- Syphilis can be treated with antibiotics.
- Both partners must be treated before the baby is born.
- After delivery, the newborn baby must be treated.

Prevention of syphilis

- Young people must abstain from sexual contact _and delay sexual relations for as long as possible.
- One should have a sexual relationship with one uninfected partner. The risk of acquiring STIs increases with the <u>number of partners over a lifetime</u>
- One should use a condom correctly and consistently to prevent and control other STIs.

- . If one has been diagnosed with syphilis, one has the responsibility to notify all recent sex partners and urge them to get a checkup.
- One should complete the full course of medication prescribed.
- One can only ensure that the infection has been cured after a follow-up test to treatment is negative
- while being treated for an STI one must avoid all sexual activity and abstain from alcohol..

Genital Warts

Genital warts are caused by human papillomavirus (HPV), a virus related to the virus that causes common skin warts.

Certain high-risk types of HPV are thought to <u>cause cancer of the cervix</u>(mouth of uterus) and other genital cancers.

- Genital warts usually first appear as small, hard painless lumps in the vaginal area, on the penis, or around the anus.
- The warts multiply quickly and develop into a fleshy, <u>cauliflower-like appearance</u>.
- Thee warts may reduce the vaginal opening causing delay in delivery of the baby resulting in fetal distress.
- Vaginal warts may cause tears during delivery as the female structures fail to stretch to allow for delivery of the baby.
- Genital warts may cause poor and slow healing of bruises after deliver.

- Genital warts make control of haemorrhage difficult after delivery. A baby born to a mother with the warts can contract the virus.

- Genital warts on the head of the penis and under the foreskin in men can make sexual activity difficult and painful.

- The warts may bleed during sexual activity increasing the chances of viral transmission to sexual partner.

- Genital warts can be treated with ointment applied to the growth.

- The warts can be treated by specialist doctors in a procedure called (freezing) in which extremely cold rods are applied to the growth.

- Very large warts can be removed surgically or by burning them,(cauterization) with specialist equipment.
- Antiretroviral drugs can be used to prevent recurrence of the growth. Both partners must be treated.

Prevention

- HPV vaccine can be given to teenagers from 13-15 years to prevent the viral infection.
- Young adolescence are advised to delay engaging in sexual activity and when they become sexually active, they are advised to have one sexual partner.
- It is advisable to use a condom always for sexual activity.

Gonorrhoea

This is a sexually transmitted infection caused by gonococci bacteria.

- The most common symptoms of gonorrhoea are a pus-like discharge from the vagina or penis.
- The infected individual has pain or difficulty in passing urine.
- The most common and serious complications of gonorrhoea is blockage of fallopian tubes in women causing ectopic pregnancy and infertility.
- In men gonorrhoea may cause blockage of the epidydimus causing infertility.
- Abscesses can form in the groins(bubos) in both men and women, in between the labia and in glands in

women and around the anus for both men and women.

- Oral gonococcal infection and gonococcal tonsilitis can occur in those who practice oral sex

- Gonorrhoea can be treated with antibiotics. It is important that one takes the full course of antibiotics

- The partner must be treated too.

- An infected mother can pass the infection to her newborn baby at birth causing neonatal gonococcus sore eyes (opthalmia neonatorum) in which a baby's eyes discharges pus soon after birth.

Trichomoniasis

This is infection of the genital tract by the organism trichomonas Vaginalis.

- The infected female has large amounts of offensive greenish, yellowish frothy vaginal discharge.
- The labia are swollen.
- The vaginal walls are swollen(vaginitis), and have reddish spots. The vulva and inner thighs are sore.
- The infected person has pain when passing urine (dysuria)
- The urethra is swollen(,urethritis),
- The bladder can be swollen,(cystitis).
- One has pain during sexual intercourse(dyspareunia).

- Trichomoniasis often occurs at the same time with gonorrhoea.
- Males have a pus discharge from their urethras.
- There is lower abdominal pain and pain on passing urine (dysuria).
- In males the prostate can be swollen(prostatitis).
- It is important that one consults health personnel for treatment.

Prevention of the infection

Both partners must exercise high standards of cleanliness and must wash genitals after intercourse.

- The use of a condom prevents transmission of infection from one partner to the other.

Scabies

- Scabies, pubic lice, ringworm are spread through close contact especially where there is poor hygiene.
- It is important to regularly shave pubic hair to enable improved hygiene and prevent lice, scabies, and ringworm.

Thrush

This is a fungal infection that causes vulval irritation and a watery offensive, milky curds, cheesy discharge from the vagina.

- In men, milky curds can be seen under the foreskin.
- There is an itchy watery offensive discharge from the penis.

- The vulval area is itchy and one feels like scratching all the time.
- There is severe discomfort when touching the vulva and when passing urine.
- The infection may be common in pregnancy and in women with diabetes and HIV infection.
- In males there is itchiness of the urethra and pain and soreness when passing urine.
- One should seek medical treatment and must exercise high standards of hygiene.
- One should wear pants with cotton gusset, or walk around without knickers
- Oral and anal sex are known sources of thrush.

- **Use of a condom is advised.**

Chapter 5

THE HUMAN-IMMUNO DEFIENCY VIRAL (HIV) INFECTION AND ACQUIRED IMMUNO-DEFICIENCY SYNDROME (AIDS)

One of the most dreaded sexually transmitted diseases is HIV infection. It is important that women are aware of how this disease impacts on their lives.

- The Human-Immuno Defiency Virus (HIV) is mainly spread through sexual intercourse between men and women or between men in homosexual relationships.

- There is infection through blood transfusion, needle pricks and congenital infection passed on from infected parents.

- It is important that one is awareness of the simple signs of HIV infection.

- Any young man who catches flues, chills, coughs and sore throats every now and then and suffers from malaria even in the dry heat of the hot seasons is suspicious.

- Thrush in the mouth of an adult should be suspect. Swollen lymph nodes behind the ears are signs of infection

- The surest way for anyone to know if their partner is a safe partner is to <u>TAKE AN HIV TEST</u> when you think you are in love and before you have an unprotected sexual activity!

- Once one is infected, one's sexual partner is likely to be infected if precautions to protect oneself are not taken.
- It may take months or years before one feels unwell depending on how strong the infecting virus is and how healthy the infected individual is.
- An infected person who has not yet developed the disease may look well and have no symptoms. The presence of the virus can be detected through a laboratory test and quick tests done by special health institutions. Once an individual has the virus in their system, it does not go away because *any drugs known to date cannot kill the virus*.

- Individuals infected by the virus will usually or may have experienced other sexually transmitted diseases like thrush of the genitals, genital warts, boils in the groins and the genital parts, genital sores and genital discharge of varying types(thick creamy pus of gonorrhea usually combined with syphilis, or thin watery pus or milky curds .

- Urinary tract infection characterized by lower abdominal pain and discomfort and pain on passing urine is also common in HIV infection.

AIDS (Acquired Immuno-Deficiency Syndrome)

- When an HIV infected person begins to feel and show signs of ill health, the initial stages of the presence of disease, Aids, may present like flue.
- One feels weak, feverish, and feels hot and cold. One may have a headache.
- There is profuse sweating at night and a general feeling of ill health. These symptoms may repeat themselves several times and quite frequently.
- As the illness progresses, the blood *falls short of its major components* like iron resulting in a person looking pale, breathless, weak and frail. Every system of the body is affected.

The Circulatory System

- The *heart is weakened*. One feels breathless at slight effort.
- The blood flow is affected and feet swell. If bleeding occurs, such as in minor injury, surgery, and tooth extraction, it becomes very difficult to control because the clotting factors are diminished

The Immune System

Cells that protect against diseases (Antibodies) cannot control these symptoms resulting in the body being attacked by any bacteria or virus that comes by (opportunistic infections) because the body can no longer protect itself. The individual becomes sickly.

The Respiratory System

- *Bacterial infections* like *pneumonia, and tuberculosis* occur repeatedly. These two conditions cause severe chest pain and breathlessness, and a persistent cough.
- The lungs may be filled with fluid preventing them from taking in oxygen and expanding as expected in the process of breathing.
- Drugs given to treat tuberculosis and pneumonia offer a temporary relief and do not completely heal the lungs, which remain with permanent scars and are likely to get re-infected.

The Digestive system

- The *digestive system is inflamed.* The lips become swollen and the skin pills off leaving blisters and raw flesh.
- The mouth may have a white coating (thrush), which is more marked in the morning when one wakes up. When one brushes or cleans the mouth of the white milk curds scabs of thrush, the mucous membrane of the mouth peels off leaving red, raw and sore flesh exposed. One has difficulty chewing their food as the mouth is sore.
- The rest of the digestive system is swollen and irritable and fails to digest food or absorb it resulting in loss of appetite, *indigestion and diarrhoea,* vomiting and loss of weight.

The Nervous System

- The thin layer of tissue that covers the brain may become swollen, a condition known as *meningitis*.
- One suffers from severe persistent headaches that are very uncomfortable and causes one to become irritable.
- Meningitis may cause *mental confusion, blindness, loss of hearing, and stroke.*

The Skin

- The *skin becomes rough.* A stubborn rash may appear on the face and body.
- One may have boils on any part of the body.
- A typical skin reaction of blisters due to the viral poison (herpes) may appear on

any part of the body such as the face, abdomen, back or thighs.

- Wounds fail to heal.
- The hair becomes thin, straight and unhealthy like that of a malnourished child.
- Once the virus is in the body, it is there to stay. One may feel strong for a while but this is a temporary relief. <u>AIDS HAS NO CURE!</u> Antiretroviral drugs give a temporary feeling of well being but do not kill the virus.
- <u>Every member of society has a responsibility to stop the spread of the virus.</u>
- AIDS is a long-term disease. One may suffer from ill health for many years before one succumbs to the disease.

- Aids_affects work, and yet it is very expensive to live with the disease.
- One has to be seen regularly by the doctor and buy expensive drugs.
- One has to eat well too to keep healthy. A poor diet can only make one deteriorate faster. One should eat three meals a day and snacks in between meals. Eat vitamin supplements and plenty of fruit and vegetables.
- One can live with the disease if they report early to health personnel and are commenced on antiretroviral treatment. This means that one has to take their medication as instructed and continue to go for reviews.
- More potent antiretroviral drugs are continuously being discovered to enable

infected persons to live as normal a life as possible but caution must be taken that one adheres to the advice they get from health personnel.

- Use a condom all the time. Infecting another person deliberately is an offense.
- Have one sexual partner

Chapter 6

MALE CIRCUMCISION

This is a surgical procedure to remove the foreskin covering the end of the penis. Circumcision is reported from the Biblical days of the Israelites and has been associated with Jewish and Muslim religions. Circumcision is also fairly common among the English.

Why should one be circumcised?

- Bacteria and viruses are known to hide under the moist foreskin where these micro-organisms (germs) grow and find their way into the body through bruises during sexual intercourse.

- This is more so especially where one does not wash after sexual intercourse.

- While washing reduces the population of micro-organisms under the fore skin, it may not completely clear the microorganisms depending on the thoroughness of the washing.

What are proven advantages of circumcision?

Male circumcision or the surgical removal of the foreskin in men <u>does not prevent</u> sexually transmitted diseases <u>but limits infection by at least 60%</u>.

- Where there is a foreskin many micro-organisms will sit and multiply in the skin fold but surgery makes the skin tough and easy to wash.
- The advantages of circumcision are that circumcision coupled with washing after

sexual intercourse removes the bulk of micro-organisms on the man. The micro-organisms have nowhere to hide and multiply.

- Circumcised men have a reduced risk of carrying human papillomavirus that causes cancer of the cervix in their partners.
- Circumcised men also have a reduced risk of acquiring chancroid and syphilis and other sexually transmitted diseases.
- In this era of HIV, male circumcision is associated with a reduced risk of HIV infection.

When is the best time for one to be circumcised?

Circumcision is a choice that one can make at any time in life. Circumcision should be an informed decision that one makes as a precaution for prevention of sexually transmitted diseases as scientific research knowledge has now revealed.

- In some cultures though, some parents make this choice for their children for cultural and religious reasons.
- Some communities that practice circumcision prefer that it is done within the first week of birth, others consider circumcision as a ritual that marks the transition of a young man into a man.
- Circumcision can therefore be done at any age.

What are the side effects of circumcision?

- There is the obvious wound complications especially pain and sometimes swelling, haemorrhage and infection.
- The risk of pain is reported to be similar to that of an injection. These side effects are very minimal especially where the operation has been done by health professionals using sterile equipment and antibiotics.

How soon after circumcision can one resume sexual activity?

- Like any operation one needs to rest after operation to prevent swelling and haemorrhage and must observe good hygiene to prevent infection.

- It is best to wait for at least six weeks before resuming sexual activity to prevent haemorrhage, bruising and infection.

- Avoid tight underwear and wear loose airy underwear.

- Avoid excessive activity like walking long distances, golf, jogging and sprinting until one is completely healed.

Is one completely free from sexually transmitted infections after circumcision?

- One is never completely free from contracting a disease. Micro-organisms may penetrate through bruises during the sexual act but a large percentage of the germs cannot enter one's body.

- The reported success of circumcision in preventing sexually transmitted diseases is not a licence for reckless behaviours.
- One must still be responsible and stick to one sexual partner.

Does circumcision alter sensation and sexual enjoyment?

- The most sensitive part of the man, the head or glans penis is not tempered with during circumcision.
- Circumcised men and their partners therefore enjoy their sexual relationship without fear of reduced sensation.

Chapter 7

DAD: CARE OF YOUR PREGNANT SPOUSE

Unless a man understands the changes that are taking place inside his partner as a result of pregnancy, he may not be able to support her adequately. It is important to understand that when a woman is pregnant she needs extra care remembering that a pregnant woman is performing a noble task, that of giving life to a new human being.

• Every man desires to have a healthy family. Early pregnancy is the time to lay foundations for a healthy family.

- Ensure that your spouse is attended to and examined by health personnel in the first three months of pregnancy.

- Accompany your spouse to see health personnel if she has headaches, backache or any unusual complaints. It is important that health problems are attended to early before major complications set in.

- You are encouraged to be present as health personnel advise on the health of your spouse as this information assists you in caring for your spouse.

- Make preparations for the arrival of the baby early and start shopping for the baby early. It is expensive to buy all baby requirements after the baby is born.

General Spousal Care

- It is important to note that a woman needs love more than anything else.
- Give your spouse those small things that she desires most during this period. It is small things that matter in a relationship. In early pregnancy your spouse may not be comfortable with certain foods. Encourage her to eat fruit, dry biscuits, and any foods she can tolerate. A sweet cup of tea before your spouse gets out of bed may reduce nausea and vomiting.
- If your spouse has problems keeping food down, and is continuously vomiting, take her to health personnel as soon as possible before she becomes dehydrated.

110

- Provide a well balanced diet to your spouse to promote good health throughout pregnancy and after delivery. A healthy mother has high chances of having a healthy baby. A healthy mother has high chances of carrying a baby who develops well, has a good weight at birth and is well protected against diseases.

- Ensure that your spouse has adequate time to rest to prevent swelling of feet, and to encourage a good flow of blood to the heart, brain, kidneys and to the growing baby.

- A woman gets time to rest if the partner helps her with household chores and you take over the difficult jobs in the home.

- Quickly take your spouse to the hospital if she bleeds while pregnant. Bleeding in pregnancy puts the lives of both mother and baby in danger.

- Quickly get your spouse to the hospital or health personnel if she feels tired or she feels her heart beat fast as if she is frightened (palpitations).

- Your partner must be seen by health personnel as soon as possible if her feet swell, her fingers and face look swollen, if she complains of dizziness or poor vision.

- Do not buy your spouse off- the- counter medications. She must be seen by health personnel who will decide if certain medicines can be taken by a pregnant woman.

Can we continue to have Sexual Relations when my partner is pregnant?

- It is advisable that you continue with sexual relationships until the day your spouse goes into labour. You need to use sexual positions that ensure that your spouse is comfortable and do not cause pressure on your spouse's abdomen or cause her backache.
  You can approach from the back, you can both kneel, you can sit your spouse on your lap, your wife can take the top position and sits astride you as you lie facing up.

- Sexual intercourse in pregnancy does not hurt the baby in any way because the baby lies far away from the vagina. The mouth of the uterus, the cervix, is closed and plugged with a thick plug of firm mucus. Semen does not get to the baby in any way; it always flows out after a sexual act!

- You are advised against engaging in extra marital relationships (small houses)! This is a source of sexually transmitted diseases including HIV. Small houses are a source of marital instability and unhappiness. Please resist that temptation. Stick to your one partner for the sake of your health and happiness and that of your family.

What you can do to assist your spouse while in labour

- On the day your spouse goes into labour please be there to support her. Make arrangements in advance to take leave from work and be present when your baby is born.

- Your presence calms your spouse and dispels undue anxieties because you can chat and she has someone close to her that she relates to in a special way.

- You can massage her back to relieve backache. You should be familiar with this activity if you attend antenatal classes with your spouse.

- You can fetch her ice-cubes, sips of water as she feels very hot and dry

- You can wipe her face, chest and back with a wet face flannel to cool her

- You can encourage her to take deep breaths as the labour pains come

- You can chat with her in between contractions (labour pains).

115

When the baby is delivered:

- You can be offered to cut the umbilical cord, or you can ask to do that. This is known to build a special relationship with your newly born baby

Help at Home:

- Help your partner with house chores to give her time to rest and recover
- Assist with baby care, bathing and dressing the baby, laundry and anything that requires to be done
- Ensure that your partner has good food, fruit and vegetables, fresh fruit juices. A good diet helps your spouse to recover quickly.

When can you resume sexual activity?

- It is not advisable for your partner to live with a relative far away. It is <u>not possible</u> to bond with your new baby or show your love fully when you are separated from your partner. Your spouse should stay close to you.

- You can resume sexual activity as soon as your spouse stops bleeding after delivery. This is usually after two to three weeks. Your partner may have some discomfort if she had an episiotomy (a cut on the opening of the birth canal to ease delivery of the baby). You need to be as gentle as possible initially. You may need to adopt sexual positions you used in pregnancy for a while if your partner was delivered by Caesarean Section.

- Prevent another pregnancy too soon. Use a condom or encourage your partner to use contraception soon after delivery. Health personnel will provide you with information on suitable contraceptives available.

Chapter 8

IMPOTENCE

What is impotence?

This is failure for a man to be aroused, attain and sustain erection for normal coitus.

What age group is affected by this problem?

- Young men may have impotence. This is called primary erectile dysfunction which is failure to have ever attained an erection at any time in one's life.

- Primary erectile dysfunction is usually caused by fear of intimacy in young people that have been exposed to bad experiences or brought up in violent environments or abused sexually or physically.

- Primary erectile dysfunction can be caused by lack of close relationships and close friends.

- Fear of the sexual act can occur if one does not have enough information about the sexual organs. There is no need for one to have poor sexual information as this is readily available at your nearest health centre, and your GP.

- Young people may be overly anxious and depressed or just feeling low due to some events in one's social life which may affect the sexual function of the individual.

- If one is feeling guilty about something this can also interfere with sexual function. If there is disharmony in one's relationship and resentment this may cause erectile dysfunction.

Mature people may have more erectile dysfunction than young people.

- Fatigue may cause erectile failure. The average man needs to rest and relax before engaging in sexual activity.
- Diseases such as diabetes, heart, high blood pressure sexually transmitted diseases, alcoholism, and diseases of the thyroid cause a general muscular weakness that may affect erection.
- People who are dependent on strong drugs may have impotence.
- Swelling of the genital organs due to sexually transmitted infections may

cause low desire for sexual activity and impotence.

- Injury such as bruising of genital organs and fear of pain may cause lack of sexual desire and lack of erection.

- Backache and any injury affecting the brain, spine, muscles and nerves of the legs may result in erectile failure.

- In aging, erection is maintained but there may be a problem in ejaculation due to reduced amounts of semen as the seminal glands reduce in size and function.

- Hidden causes like enlarged prostate gland may cause impotence.

People on long term treatment for hypertension, epilepsy, asthma, people on drugs that enhance performances, steroids and strong pain relief may have erectile dysfunction.

Secondary erectile dysfunction

Secondary erectile dysfunction is failure to complete successful sexual intercourse because of inability to attain or maintain erection.

- Poor flow of the male hormone, testosterone, causes secondary erectile dysfunction
- .Anxiety, fear of failure to perform to the satisfaction of a partner as well as desire to please partner may cause erectile dysfunction.
- Demand for performance from a partner can cause secondary erectile dysfunction.

- Excessive consumption of alcohol deflates one's performance.

It is important for partners to feel free to express their sexual problems with each other. If one has a problem, it is important to express it to health personnel so that possible causes are explored and one can be assisted to work out a way forward.

Managing erectile problems

There are many myths and beliefs associated with erectile dysfunction.

- It is important to share one's problem with one's partner so that she understands the problem.
- It helps for the couple to visit the doctor together. Health personnel will ask

many questions about one's ife and sexual life to obtain information that could have caused the problem.

- A thorough examination to investigate any obvious problems like tumours and swelling of the genitals is done.
- Laboratory tests will be done to exclude diabetes, thyroid disease, and determine testosterone levels.

Can one cure low sexual drive by using alternative medicines, herbs and additives to foods?

- Use of various herbal powders, animal horn powders in food or beer has no proven positive effect in treating low sexual drive.

Care must be taken that one does not eat poisonous preparations that can cause kidney problems and harm other parts of the body.

- High salt intake and high intake of cheese and spices too have no proven positive effect on one's sexual drive.
- There are proven ways of managing low sexual drive and impotence and it is advisable to seek professional help.

Sexual Technique

- Erectile problems may be corrected by engaging in a lengthy foreplay before the actual sexual act.
- Lengthy foreplay is also good for one's partner as women often feel hurried by

their partners before they are ready for the act.

- Practicing a three stage technique of a sexual act starting with an emphasis on touching and caressing one's partner, followed by oral foreplay or kissing, then lastly genital pleasuring when both partners are ready stimulates sexual desire and hormone production that maintains erection.

- Non- demanding, free flowing or automatic coitus usually occurs where both partners are ready.

- It helps to talk about marital problems and resolve them and iron out your differences before engaging in a sexual activity,

- A couple can see a marriage counselor or psychologist for help if the above measures do not help you.

Premature ejaculation
Failure to withhold ejaculation long enough until one's partner is ready occurs quite often. This is more so because men are ready to ejaculate within a short time.

- Women take a lot longer to be aroused and to reach orgasm and may be frustrated if the partner is done before they are ready.
- It is important that a man learns to withhold ejaculation until the partner is ready.

- Premature ejaculation may occur because of fear of failure, fear of making the partner pregnant, and lack of experience.
- Other causes of premature ejaculation are prolonged intervals before sexual intercourse, and inflammatory conditions such as swollen prostate gland (prostatitis).
- Managing premature ejaculation should include practicing to stop sexual activity as soon as the urge to ejaculate comes and starting once more in order to delay ejaculation.

Failure to ejaculate
This is failure to achieve ejaculation of semen during a sexual act.

- Failure to ejaculate can be associated with high levels of anxiety and poor relaxation.
- Other causes of failure to ejaculate are diabetes, and drugs for treatment of various long term illnesses. Prolonged foreplay stimulates one and may enable ejaculation when one is ready.
- Low sex drive may progress to become impotence. There may not be any problem with erection or orgasm, or loss of pleasure but there could be an underlying psychological problem or low hormonal levels.
- Using varying sexual positions may improve sex drive.

Chapter 9

PROBLEMS AND TUMOURS OF THE GENITAL ORGANS

1.Hydrocele

This is collection of fluid in the scrotum, the sac that contains and holds the testes.

Where does the fluid come from?

- This fluid is not a bad spell. The fluid is not caused by the types of food one eats.
- The fluid oozes from the blood vessels that supply the scrotum and collects in between layers of tissue that form the scrotal sac which protects testes.

How does a hydrocele affect a person?

- This condition can be depressing and causes low morale, embarrassment and lack of confidence.

- One may prefer to isolate themselves to avoid this embarrassment. One may need to wear larger size trousers or wear a jacket all the time to conceal the abnormal bulge between legs. Other people's way of walking (gait) is also affected.

- Hydrocele affects sexual relations. Where the hydrocele is very large, the penis is pulled inside the bulge and this causes problems in emptying the bladder.

- Apart from causing a poor urine stream resulting in one messing themselves when emptying the bladder, a hydrocele can also cause dribbling of urine requiring that one wears a pad to receive the dribble.

How can it be managed?

- Once you realize that your scrotum is getting unusually large on one side or all round, see health personnel immediately for help.
- There is no need to carry this heavy awkward bulge around. A hydrocele can be drained and one regains their normal shape of the male structures again.
- Sometimes the fluid keeps on coming back and collecting in which case the doctors may decide to perform some surgery to reduce the size of the sac and prevent further collection of fluid.

- After surgery, one needs to rest to prevent swelling.
- Normal sexual relationships can be resumed as soon as one heals and is pain free.

2. Enlarged Prostate Gland

What is a prostate gland?

The prostate gland lies below the bladder of men and surrounds the urethra or urine passage.

What is the function of the prostate gland?

The prostate gland produces large amounts of semen discharged by a man during sexual intercourse. Semen allows the male seed to swim easily to reach the female egg for possible fertilization. Semen is also produced by the testes or men's balls that are in the scrotum and seminal vesicles that lie on the sides of the bladder slightly above the prostate gland.

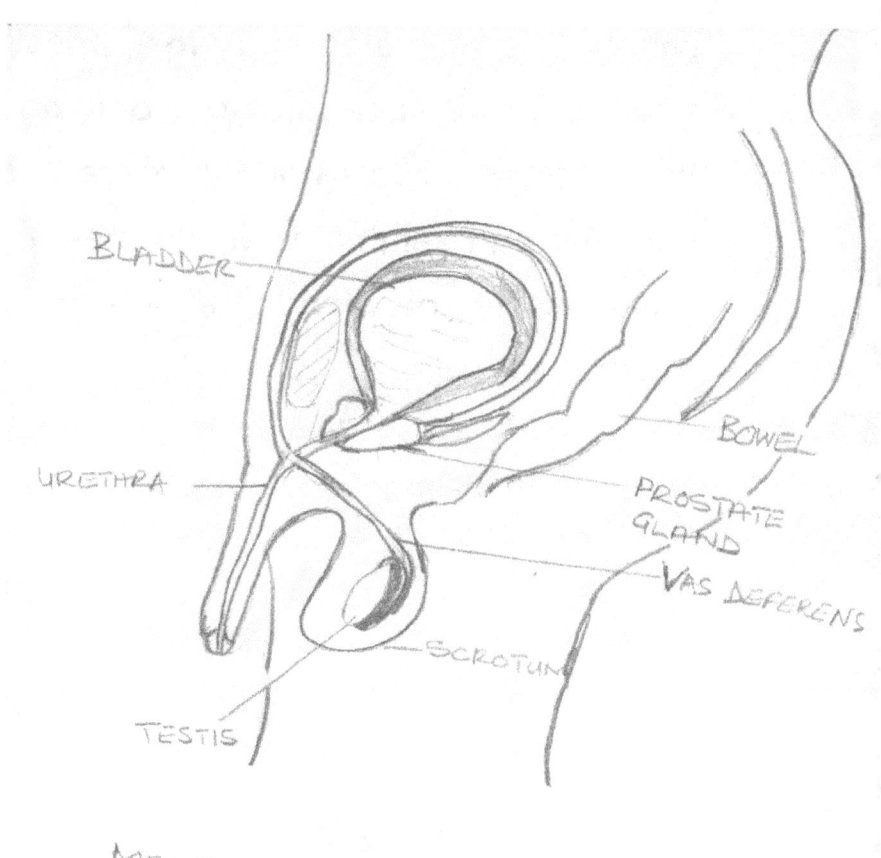

BLADDER

URETHRA

BOWEL

PROSTATE
GLAND

VAS DEFERENS

SCROTUM

TESTIS

MALE ORGANS

What happens when the prostate gland is enlarged?

The prostate gland in some men has a tendency to increase in size with age. As the prostate gland grows, it affects one's waterworks in various ways as follows:

- The prostate gland pushes inwards towards the urethra reducing the opening of the urethra as it grows. It pushes upwards towards the bladder, affecting effective empting of the bladder, causing a poor stream and reducing the ability of the bladder to hold normal amounts of urine.

One feels the urge to pass urine every now and then (frequency) because the pressure of the growing prostate limits

137

the amount of urine the bladder can hold.

- The prostate gland pushes outwards towards the bowel and may cause constipation.
- As it pushes upwards and in advanced cases, the enlarged prostate gland causes problems in emptying the bladder. One may feel discomfort or pain when emptying the bladder (dysuria). One may fail to completely empty the bladder so that there is always stagnant urine in the bladder (residual urine) attracting germs that multiply in the bladder causing bladder in swelling and irritation (cystitis). The urine may have a nasty smell and a dark color because of the infection.

- Sometimes the prostate gland grows so big that one fails to pass urine (retention of urine), a very uncomfortable condition in which the bladder may stretch towards the abdomen causing swelling of the abdomen.

How is the enlarged prostate gland managed?

- If one has retention of urine, a tube (bladder catheter) passed through the urethra is used to drain the urine from the bladder. One may have to have this tube in the bladder for a while as a temporary measure while waiting for surgery. One may have a bag to this bladder tube that one must empty whenever it is full.

- The bladder tube (catheter) is changed at specific periods to prevent further infection. If one's urine system has infection, it is treated and one is advised to have surgery.
- One is advised to drink lots of water to clear the bladder infection.
- Surgery is the answer to an enlarged prostate. The doctor will explain the details of the surgery and one has an opportunity to ask relevant questions that may be worrying one.
- One method of surgery that the doctor may suggest is (TURP) Transurethral prostatectomy in which the doctor reduces the size of the prostate gland by scrapping out fragments of the prostate gland through the urethra.

- The prostate fragments are sent to the laboratory to exclude cancer of the prostate. Cancer of the prostate is the commonest cancer in men.

- The doctor will share the laboratory results with you and advise you on your health. After the operation, one has to drink lots of fluids until the urine is clear.

- One must also rest for at least six weeks to three months. One must avoid activity like sports, golf, walking for long distances, jogging until one feels completely healed as such activities may cause bleeding and backache.

Can one have normal sexual relationships after surgery of the prostate?

There is no known reason why a man who has had a TURP should not be able to enjoy normal sexual relationships.

Can one father a child after a TURP?

- One can father many children after a TURP because the prostate gland does not produce the male seed.
- The prostate gland produces semen. The amounts of semen from the prostate may be reduced after TURP but there are other organs that produce semen.
- TURP is done very far away from the testes which produce the male seed. Male fertility is therefore not affected by this operation.

3. Cancers

The most common cancer in men is cancer of the prostate. It is important that from the age of forty men have an annual check up to exclude enlarged prostate and cancer of the prostate.

Who is likely to get cancer of the prostate?

Cancer of the prostate can affect any man especially from the age of forty. It is therefore wise that every man have a regular screening for cancer of the prostate from age forty onwards.

How may one feel?

In the early stages one may not have any symptoms. As the cancer progresses, one may experience progressive backache and lower abdominal pain. One may have constipation and problems with emptying of the bladder.

How is a diagnosis made?

Diagnosis is made through laboratory tests. Most cancers of the prostate are diagnosed when one has prostatectomy and prostate tissue is sent to the laboratory.

A scan is usually done especially where one has symptoms.

Management of cancers

Management depends on the extent of the cancer. Surgery may be done in early cancer followed by chemotherapy or drugs that destroy cancer cells. Chemotherapy may be combined with radiotherapy. The doctor will discuss the suitable management with each individual.

Chapter 10

SMOCKING

So you smoke? Smoking is a habit learnt and nurtured by an

individual for reasons best known to the individual. Smoking usually starts at adolescence in a bid to be noticed, to win friends, to appear cool and different and out of curiosity.

Excuses for smoking

Adult smokers come up with many lame excuses for perpetuating their bad habit of smoking. A smoker may regard his bad habit as a way of 'socializing', but the truth is that smoking is at the expense of one's health.

A smoker may call the habit a means to reduce boredom, but the smoker is slowly destroying his lungs and shortening his life.

Some smokers think that smoking helps in reduction of nervousness and bolsters courage to speak and strength to work. All these excuses are false. This is called addiction. Cigarettes contain a substance or poison called nicotine.

A smoker's body will crave for more nicotine once one is hooked to smoking. Smokers think puffing away a cigarette heats up the body on a cold day. This too is false. None of the above excuses are true.

The fact is that smoke forms a sticky tarry paste on lung tissue weakening the lung tissue.

Facts about smoking

- Nicotine is habit forming. A smoker must smoke to keep the levels of nicotine in one's body high.

- Nicotine gives a hangover or craving for more smoking. Once hooked to nicotine one craves for more and slowly one cannot do without it. Smoking is therefore habit forming. Once one starts smoking, there is a tendency to continue smoking because the body craves for more and more nicotine.

- Smoking gives one a false feeling of satisfaction and yet it imprisons a person and ties the person down to smoking.

- Smoke is absorbed into the body tissues so that one's body and all body fluids like saliva, urine, sweat, smell of cigarettes. A smoker's clothes smell of cigarettes even after washing them.

- The smoke coats one's teeth and they lose their luster. Teeth are stained into varied shades of grey that no toothpaste can completely remove. The lips, tongue and mouth are coated grey.

- A smoker's breath has strong cigarette smell making close ups and whispers very unpleasant even after using smokers toothpaste!

- Smoke coats lung tissue like oily tar reducing the lungs' ability to absorb fresh air. That is the beginning of lung diseases and breathing problems that are likely

- to end your life! Smoking and health

- Smoking reduces absorption of air by lung tissue thus reducing oxygen circulation in the body. The smoke weakens lung tissue and causes a lingering, wet, loud cough, chronic bronchitis.

- A smoker has increased chances of suffering from lung infections such as pneumonias, tuberculosis, cancer of the lungs and lung collapse.

- Smoking causes narrowing and hardening of blood vessels causing high blood pressure. Narrowing of

blood vessels that supply the heart slows down supply of blood to the heart tissue increasing the chances of heart failure.

- Smoking has the risk of fires. A cigarette stub left burning can destroy everything one has worked for all his life, other people's properties, vegetation and even lives!

Passive smoking

Smokers tend to be insensitive of others' preferences. Puffing away cigarette smoke, in a crowded place, in the presence of babies and children, wife, friends, in a pub room,

forces everyone within reach to inhale the smoke. This is forcing everyone within the reach of the smoke to be a passive smoker.

Passive smoking is more dangerous than active smoking because active smokers exhale the smoke while passive smokers keep the smoke deep in their lungs.

It is extremely selfish to make other people uncomfortable

through one's bad habits. Cigarette smoke can cause asthmatic

attack and heart attack in bystanders or members of the family.

If a smoker cares about other people, his family included, then

he must do everybody a favor and smoke outside the house

and away from the general public.

Smoking and pregnancy

Smoking narrows blood vessels and therefore reduces blood flow to the placenta, a structure attached to the mother's blood system and connected to the baby by the umbilical cord, whose function is feeding food and air to the unborn baby.

Reduced blood flow to the placenta reduces oxygen and nutrients to the

unborn child slowing down the growth of the unborn child.

A pregnant mother exposed to high levels of smoke can easily go into premature labor. The baby is born small for dates.

- The baby will have breathing problems at birth, and will need resuscitation at birth.
- A baby exposed to smoke everyday may develop upper respiratory diseases.
- The baby may be lost due to difficulty in breathing.
- The baby is in danger of cigarette burns.

- If as a couple you smoke, it is time you thought about the harm you are causing to your unborn child and the rest of the family!

- Smoking causes narrowing and hardening of blood vessels causing high blood pressure.

Narrowing of blood vessels that supply the heart slows down supply of blood to the heart tissue increasing the chances of heart failure.

Smoking has the risk of fires.

A cigarette stub left burning can destroy everything one has worked for all his life, other people's properties, vegetation and even lives! Passive smoking Smokers tend to be insensitive of others' preferences. Puffing away cigarette smoke, in a crowded place, in the presence of babies and children, wife, friends, fellow passengers in a bus, in a plane or room, forces everyone within reach to inhale the smoke.

It is extremely selfish to force everyone within your reach of the smoke to be a passive smoker.

Passive smoking is more dangerous than active smoking because active smokers exhale the smoke while passive smokers keep the smoke deep in their lungs.

It is extremely selfish to make other people uncomfortable through one's bad habits.

- Cigarette smoke can cause asthmatic attack and heart attack in bystanders or members of the family.

If you care about other people, your family included, then you must do everybody a favour and smoke outside the house and away from the general public.

Smoking and pregnancy

Smoking narrows blood vessels and therefore reduces blood flow to the

placenta, a structure attached to the mother's blood system and connected to the baby by the umbilical cord, whose function is feeding food and air to the unborn baby.

- Reduced blood flow to the placenta reduces oxygen and nutrients to the unborn child slowing down the growth of the unborn child.

- A pregnant mother exposed to high levels of smoke can easily go into premature labour.
- The baby is born small for dates.
- The baby will have breathing problems at birth, and will need resuscitation at birth.
- A baby exposed to smoke everyday may develop upper respiratory diseases.
- The baby may be lost due to difficulty in breathing. The baby is in danger of cigarette burns.
- If as a couple you smoke, it is time you thought about the harm you are causing to your unborn child and the rest of the family!

Reasons for quitting smoking

- **Smoking kills! That is a true fact. You shorten your life by many years.**
- **Smoking is expensive. There are better things to do with the money you spend on cigarettes.**
- **If you saved all the money you spend on cigarettes per month you could buy many loaves of bread for orphans!**
- **There is nothing to gain from smoking; one merely burns money and burns life away.**

How to stop smoking

The decision to stop smoking is entirely yours! Once you make up your mind that you want to stop smoking:

- Throw away everything that reminds you of a cigarette such as a cigarette lighter, ashtray and clear your garden or apartment of cigarette stubs.
- Don't buy cigarettes.
- Don't ask anybody, stranger of friend for a cigarette.
- Don't accept an offer of a cigarette.
- Tell all your friends that you have stopped smoking.
- Replace a cigarette with an apple, a sweet or snacks, peanuts etc.
- You can purchase smoke cessation patches from your pharmacy.

Chapter11

EXERCISE AND MEN

Your health is your responsibility!

Do you like the way you look in the mirror or on pictures?

Do you look like you have a second chin?

Is your belly falling onto your thighs?

Do you find it difficult to bend over because the belly is in the way?

Do you feel breathless when walking or after doing a small chore?

Are you huffing and puffing like an old steam engine when you walk?

Do you feel aches and pains in your joints?

Are you tipping your bathroom scales?

Are your clothes getting tight?

Is your belly threatening to pop out of your shirt? Have you bought clothes one size larger than before?

Is your sex life dying or dead?

If your answer is yes to some or all the above questions you need to get out of your recliner chair and join the gym for a healthy life. Lose that extra baggage you don't need it!

Big or overweight is not good living or comfort.

Overweight is living dangerously.

Why is excessive weight bad for you?

- It strains your heart.
- It raises your Blood pressure,
- It causes Diabetes,
- You can have breathing problems like asthma.

You don't need all these health problems!

Enjoy good health! Don't carry unnecessary baggage!

Do not delay starting to work on the parts of your body that are letting you down. You could join the local gym today. They will show you the relevant moves and they have got the machines to help you.   Promote your own good health!

 Enjoy a healthier life! Exercise daily and lose unnecessary weight!

What is the part of your body that lets you down?
Is it your Upper Arms?

Loose muscles that hang out of your shirt awkwardly and add on years to your actual age.

Do you feel uncomfortable wearing a sleeveless vest even in sweltering heat.

The good news is that when you decide to take up an exercise routine, consider the under arm flab a thing of the past.

You can have firm biceps and triceps by working on various machines and and gadgets that firm your arm muscles while you have fun.

Once you start on exercise, it gets into your system and becomes part of your life. The fat under your skin and in your muscle burns out and you remain with firm muscle.

Get good looking under arms that match your body and your age.

Shaping up has never been this fun.

You will love every moment you are shaping your arms!

Your Belly

This part of the body is the undoing of many people; men and women as well!

So you have handles and tyres around your waist?

Do you lift your belly to see your feet?

Do you need to stand in front of a mirror to see your pubic hair?

Does your belly sit on your thighs or flip=flop as you walk?

 Did you know that most of the big ugly rolls around your belly are all fat? There is so much room around your belly you could be carrying pounds and pounds of fat you don't need! It is unnecessary baggage! You can lose all that baggage through exercise!

Don't court health problems by keeping that excess fat on your body.

Soon your heart will be surrounded by fat restricting its ability to pump blood. Your blood vessels become coated by a fatty substance reducing their size and ability to stretch and push blood around your body. Your blood pressure rises. You become breathless and experience chest pains and headaches! You are courting major health problems! Blood flow to your lower legs becomes poor. You may have blood clotting in your lower legs! Blood clots are dangerous; they cause heart attack and stroke!

But, the good news is <u>you can get rid of the unnecessary fat!</u>   Blood clotting problems can be eased. It is a good feeling to be able to carry your body around.

 After you have lost weight you can notice that your step and your stature changes.

You will become more confident and your clothes will hang well on a trimmer body.

You will attract a lot of interest from people who never used to look at you twice. Lose weight around your belly and you will feel like new.

There is no reason why a man should carry unnecessary weight.

Your thighs

Ideally you should be able to see the formation of your thigh muscles. If your thighs have dimples and look like the skin of an orange then you should know that you are storing unnecessary fat under the skin of your thighs.

- Shape up your thighs and look attractive.

- Fit nicely into your pants/trousers

- Promote good blood flow to the rest of your leg.
- Prevent ugly varicose veins and blood clots in the lower leg.
- Fit nicely into the shoe of your choice.
- Start shaping up today, it adds more happy healthy days and months to your life.

By the nature of the physical work expected of men, it is important that men are healthy and strong.

- Pot bellies and excessive weight are unhealthy as they expose one to heart disease, high blood pressure, blood clotting and diabetes.
- A healthy man should be able to carry his weight around with ease and without feeling breathless.

The Importance of Exercise

Exercise is important for improvement of general physical fitness. Exercise burns up the stored fats and carbohydrates in the body and uses them as energy.

- Exercise enables your body to lose excess water and wastes through sweat.

- Exercise strengthens body muscles and improved body shape, stable gait and good posture.

- Exercise in general is important for movement of body joints improvement of muscle tone and prevention of stiff joints and general aches and pains.

- Exercise maintains good body balance.

- Activity makes the heart to beat harder and faster improving blood flow to all parts of the body.
- Early morning walks over a stretch of a distance improves circulation of blood around the body.
- The increase in the breathing rate during exercises draws in more air to the lungs, which expand to the maximum. The fresh air is passed onto the blood as the blood gives off carbon dioxide from muscle activity. The fresh blood prevents muscle cramps.
- Exercises tightens sagging muscles; fluid sitting in wrong places in the body is moved, fat around the belly and thighs is burnt.

- Exercise improves appetite. With good regular exercise, your appetite improves. You therefore must eat regular well balanced diet.
- Exercise improves sleep. After walking for about twenty to thirty minutes, or after a good workout at the gym, it is possible to enjoy a good nap later on in the day or a   good night's sleep.
  When is the best time to exercise?

- Exercises are more effective if done first thing in the morning or at the end of the day but before a meal.. Exercises are best done before a heavy meal. Your heart cannot cope with digesting a heavy meal as well as coping with exercise!

- It is advisable to exercise for a short period until your body adjusts to the workout. Gradually increase the time spent exercising and vary the types of exercises.
- If however you feel very tired or your health is not very good, you need to slow down.
- You should do your exercises first, have a leisurely shower or bath which is also good at toning muscles, clearing away body wastes and refreshing you before you settle down to a meal.
- A man can go jogging in one's local area or go to the local gym and to the 'Keep Fit' group exercises
- Skipping is good exercise as it moves most groups of muscles in the body.

- One can cycle or take cycling to a higher level of cycle racing.
- Dancing is a wonderful enjoyable way of keeping fit.
- Encourage your partner to join in and enjoy the advantages of exercise.
  General excuses for not exercising
  I am too old to exercise
- You need exercises in your old age than ever before. Exercises keep your joints active and prevent stiff joints.
- Exercise tone your muscles and prevent sagging of muscles and skin taking away years of ageing.
- Exercise keeps the heart and lungs healthy.
- Exercises move the bowels preventing constipation and hemorrhoids.

- Exercises promote emptying of the bladder preventing urinary infections, retention of urine and formation of bladder stones.

- After exercises, you sleep well.

  I am too busy; I have no time to exercise. I leave home early for work and come back late in the evening. I just can't fit into gym hours.

  Don't neglect your health because you are working. You must maintain good health to be able to work. Some gyms are open till late in the evening and weekends too.

  I work a lot in my garden, isn't that enough exercise?

Gardening does not exercise all your muscles. Exercise targets groups of muscles

I am recovering from an illness; wont I get ill again by exercising?

When you are ill, muscles may lose tone and become very weak. You need exercises to regain muscle tone and and general body mobility. Doctors always recommend exercise as part of the requirements for speedy recovery.

My work is very tiring; I would not have the strength to exercise everyday.

- Exercises revive you after a tiring day. You need to tone your muscles even after a busy day.

- If your work involves sitting in board rooms, sitting behind a desk, you need to move your leg muscles to promote good blood circulation and prevent blood clotting problems and varicose veins.
- Exercise refreshes your brain. The blood rush to your brain revives and activates the brain cells and makes you a sharp thinker.

  I am wheelchair bound;it is not possible to exercise
- You have a sedentary life, you need to keep your heart healthy through exercise.
- You must burn the food you eat through exercise or risk the problem of overweight, diabetes, high blood

pressure, poor blood flow and clots formation. Clots in your blood system cause heart attack or stroke.

Exercise for mature people

Mature people need to exercise to keep blood flowing smoothly, prevent clots, varicose veins and swelling of feet. Mature people need to exercise to prevent stiffness of joints and to improve mobility.

It is best to exercise every part of the body where possible. You can start with any part of the body as follows:

Sit in a straight firm chair to prevent staggering and falls which may further reduce your mobility.

The head

- Move your head from side to side five times.
- Fill your cheeks with air and slowly blow out five times.
- Move your face muscles slowly from side to side five times
- Close your eyes tightly and open five times. These exercises prevent sagging of face muscles improve the tone of face muscles especially where one is recovering from facial paralysis and make you look youthful!

The chest

It is important that your heart and lungs are kept healthy. These two organs are vital organs to life. You need healthy lungs that can take in as much air as possible when you breathe in. Your heart needs fresh blood with lots of oxygen for it to pump blood well.

- Take a deep breath through the nose and slowly breathe out. Repeat five to ten times.

Arms

Keep your arms mobile and active.

- When you walk swing your arms to keep the joints flexible.

- While sitting in the chair, raise your arms as high as you can.

- Swing your arms from side to side five times

- Wave your arms from side to side (Mexican wave)

- Shake your hands moving all your fingers

- Touch the tip of your thumb with the tip of each finger
- Make a tight fist with each hand; straighten your fingers and repeat five times
- Squeeze a tennis ball or a folded piece of cloth in each hand. Repeat for at least five minutes
- Try netball from the comfort of your chair to help improve flexibility of your whole hand.

Legs

To prevent stiffness of your leg joints you must exercise your legs!

- Every morning take a walk around your yard, around your block or down the road for at least fifteen to twenty minutes.

- While seated in a firm chair, move your legs in marching movements ten times.
- Lift your foot and move it in circular movements
- Bend your foot up and down five times and repeat with the other foot
- Move your lower leg in kicking movements five times. Repeat with the other leg
- Draw circles in the air with one foot and repeat with the other foot
- Stand up and do the marching movements while in one spot.
- If your legs are unstable you should lean on your walking stick, on a chair or against a firm table.

Chapter 12

Your Food and Your Health

To stay healthy, cut down or stop taking foods that cause problems to your health.

- Cut down on fats, starches, sugary foods and alcohol.
- Eat more fruit and vegetables for vitamins and iron that prevent diseases and boost your immune system. The relaxing thought is that you don't need to think about calories or weight gain, in fact you don't need to worry about overeating; the more you eat the better it is for your body.
- You will look younger.

- You will have regular bowel movements that prevent colonic diseases like colitis because wastes don't sit for long periods in your bowel.

- Fruit and vegetables fill your stomach quickly. There won't be need to stuff yourself with lots of starches and fats that add unnecessary stuff that your body does not need in large quantities.

- Your general health improves! You will prevent and limit minor ailments like the common cold and general body weakness or fatigue.

- You will feel healthier than ever before. The healthier you are, the more energy you have. The smooth skin makes you look younger. You will feel more confident among others. Your friends will certainly notice the glow on your skin.

- You are likely to be showered with compliments by friends and admirers. There will be a marked reduction in your health bills too!

How do fruits and vegetables cause this transformation in you?

Fruit and vegetables contain vitamins which are the source of good health.

- Fruit and vegetables contain minerals that the body needs to function well.
- Some vegetables are sources of vegetable protein that the body needs to build antibodies and other fine proteins to prevent bleeding and fight disease.

- These fine proteins are found in body fluids and inside body tissues

  Here are a few facts about the magic elements your body gains when you eat a selection of fruit and vegetables.

- Vegetables are low in fats and have no cholesterol and calories.
- Fruit and vegetables contain plenty of dietary fiber which reduce blood cholesterol and lower the risk of heart disease and heart attacks.
- Fiber reduces constipation! What an easy way to stop the straining on hard bruising stools!
- Vegetables contain folic acid which is necessary for healthy red blood cells that increase your haemoglobin and

prevent anemia. If you hemoglobin is good then you have healthy blood that attracts oxygen and your tissues stay healthy.

Asparagus has fiber that is filling and moves bowels. It also has Vit.C

Beans, lentils, black eyed beans, kidney beans pinto beans, limabeans, chick peas contain potassium and fiber and vegetable protein.

Broccoli is rich in iron and Vit.K. It is recommended for healing after surgery, long illnesses in chronic diseases and prevention of cancers

Carrots,are loaded with Vit.A essential for maintaining good eye-sight. Carrots are filling and when eaten raw contain fiber. All age groups need Vit.A more so children, the elderly and anyone whose eyesight is compromised by disease such as diabetes.

Cabbage has fiber, Vit.K, potassium, Vit C and is a multi-purpose vegetable which can be eaten raw in salads and cooked

Cauliflower is rich in Vit C essential in prevention of chronic diseases

Celery is eaten for its high fiber content.

Garlic gives a lovely aroma to food. Garlic has soothing effect on nerves and relaxes smooth muscle and by so doing lowers blood pressure

Ginger is added to dishes in cooking for its refreshing flavor. Ginger has medicinal properties. For many years women have used ginger to make medicinal teas to treat coughs and abdominal upset. Ginger flavored beverages are believed to be energizing.

Green peppers add flavor to cooking and salads. They are bulky and filling. They too have Vit.C

Lettuce and Kale. Green leafy vegetables are rich in Vit. K, calcium and iron essential in healthy blood. Your general health improves! You will prevent and limit minor ailments like the common cold and general body weakness or fatigue. You will feel healthier than ever before. The healthier you are, the more energy you have. The smooth skin you gain makes you look younger. You will feel more confident among others. Your friends will certainly notice the glow on your skin. You are likely to be showered with compliments by friends and admirers. There will be a marked reduction in your health bills too!

How do fruits and vegetables cause this transformation in you?

- Fruit and vegetables contain vitamins which are the source of good health. Fruit and vegetables contain minerals that the body needs to function well.
- Some vegetables are sources of vegetable protein that the body needs to

build antibodies and other fine proteins to prevent bleeding and fight disease. These fine proteins are found in body fluids and inside body tissues

Here are a few facts about the magic elements your body gains when you eat a selection of fruit and vegetables.

Vegetables are low in fats and have no cholesterol and calories. They contain plenty of dietary fiber which reduce blood cholesterol and lower the risk of heart disease and heart attacks. Fiber reduces constipation! What an easy way to stop the straining on hard bruising stools!

The roughage or fiber in fruit and vegetables reduces cholesterol and lowers your blood pressure.

Roughage is filling so you can replace the large amounts of starchy foods like rice, pasta, maize-meal breads with a variety of vegetables on your dinner plate.

Fruit

Fruits are low in sodium and calories. They have no cholesterol. Fruits in general contain potassium, fiber, Vit.C and Folic Acid.

Bananas, prunes, peaches apricots, melon have potassium

Dietary fiber in fruits reduces cholesterol and prevent heart disease and lower blood pressure, prevent obesity and type 2 Diabetes

Vitamin C is important for growth and repair of worn out body tissiues and wound healing, healthy teeth and gums

Folic Acid is essential for healthy blood cells and is especially needed in early pregnancy to prevent fetal abnormalities. Fruits reduces heart

disease, stroke, obesity and cancers and type 2 Diabetes. Fruits reduce risk of kidney stones and bone disease

Apples like other fruit contain Vit C, fructose and fiber. Apples refresh the mouth and have a tooth cleaning effect. Apples prevent constipation

Avocados contain an abundance of Vit.D and rich vegetable oils great for smooth skin texture and tissue health. Avocados are a versatile fruit that can be eaten on its own, as part of salad with combination with vegetables and in preparing sumptuous sandwiches.

Bananas are rich in potassium a substance essential for effective muscle action and especially good for the health of heart muscle. Contrary to the common belief that Bananas can cause constipation, they have threads which contribute to fiber essential for bowel movement and generate gas essential for bowel movement.

Grapes contain Vit C and fructose. They can be eaten as a snack, in fruit salad as a desert. Grapes can be made into grape juice, wines and can be mixed with other fruit in mixed fruit juices.

Melon, Kiwis contain Vit C and have abundance of fructose the energy giving easily absorbable fruit sugars which is less concentrated than the cane sugar and can be enjoyed in reasonable amounts by diabetics as well. Fructose is used in the preparation of artificial sweeteners. Melon seeds are packed with vegetable oils and fiber and can be eaten mixed with pumpkin seeds and other seeds and added to breads, cereals and salads.

Oranges, Lemons, Natjes are citrus fruits rich in Vitamin C and fiber. Vitamin C protects against minor respiratory problems like the common cold and allergic reactions. Vitamin C is essential for smooth skin and wound healing.

Citrus fruit peels can be used in baking recipes.

The tangy taste in all fruit has a laxative effect so constipation which can be a worrying feature in people with sedentary jobs, the elderly and those confined to bed, will be a thing of the past.

Peaches, nectarines and pears all contain Vit.C and like all fruits have a laxative effect.

Tomatoes are a very versatile fruit rich in Vit C. and potassium. Tomatoes are also a vegetable good in providing enhanced flavors in vegetable, meat and fish dishes Tomatoes can be preserved bottled, tinned, tubed as purees or dried. Fresh tomato juice is delicious.

Sweet Potatoes, white potatoes, beetroot are rich in potassium which is needed to maintain a healthy heart

Vit.B Complex is a combination of 8vitamins which often work together although each one has its specific function.

VitB1(Thiamin)Found in lentils, whole grains, yeast, nuts, seeds(sunflower),peas, beans, nuts, spinach

Vit.B2 (Riboflavin) Necessary for normal growth. It is found in cereals, spinach and broccoli

Vit.B3 (Niacin)(Nicotinic Acid). It supports chemical reactions in the body including production of energy and breaking down of fats. It promotes healthy heart function. It is found in whole wheat, peanuts, peas and beans.

Vit.B5 (Pantothenic Acid) It is required for fat breakdown and cell energy It is found in whole grains, cashew nuts, soy beans, broccoli, avocado pears, lentils

Vit.B6. (Pyridoxine). It is necessary as a source of protective proteins thus providing immunity from diseases and storage of energy. It is needed for normal nerves, production of hormones and red cells. It is found in bananas, spinach and cereals.

Vit. B7 (Biotin)

It is important in digestion of proteins, starches and fats. It is essential for healthy hair, skin and nails. It is found in yeast, strawberries, soyabeans

Vit, B9 (Folic Acid)

It is important for formation of red blood cells, and cell proteins. It is needed in early pregnancy for development of the fetus making it important for all women of the child bearing age. It is found in wheat (breads), cereals, dark green leafy vegetables like spinach. It is also found in asparagus, brewer's yeast, dates and avocado pear.

Vit.B12(Cobalamin)

It is essential for healthy cells and production of DNA, red blood cells and healthy nerves. It is mostly found in meats.

Vit C. Is essential for healthy skin. It prevents infections like common cold. It is found in beet root, carrots, broccoli, cucumber, tomato, Kale, Spinach, Cabbage, Cauliflower, celery, parsley, asparagus, Brussel sprouts, peppers, onion, ginger, strawberries, cherry, blackberry, blueberry, raspberry, citrus fruits

Vit. D is essential for healthy teeth and bones. It is important for calcium absorption essential for strong bones. Lack of Vit.D in children causes bow legs or rickets, bone deformities, osteomalacia and brittle bones. The elderly and pregnant women may require extra supplements. It is found in dairy products, seafoodsand mushrooms

Vit.K is essential for normal heart function, and clotting of blood. It is found in broccoli, Brussel sprouts, cabbage, celery, ginger, garlic, green beans, spinach, cauliflower, asparagus,

Kiwi fruit, grapes, papaya, pineapple, blackberries.

Calcium is essential for strong bones and teeth. It is found in spinach, Kale, okra, white beans, soybeans

Fluids

Drink plenty of water to wash away the wastes your body generates during exercise. Drink plenty of water to prevent kidney problems, to keep your urinary system busy and clear and prevent infections and urinary stones.

You need to drink a lot of water for smooth regular bowel movements and prevention of constipation.

All your tissues in your body need water to stay healthy. Your body needs water for healthy blood, for tears, saliva, mucus and the fluid inside each single cell that makes up the body.

Keep yourself healthy and fit and enjoy good health by living a health- conscious life.

References

Anthony,CP. et al. A Textbook of Anatomy and Physiology. CV Mosby Company, 1979 Toronto

Belloc, N. B; Breslow, L. Relationship of physical health status and health practices, *Preventive Medicine*,1972;9: 409-421

Conner, M.;Sparks, P. *The Theory of Planned Behaviour and Health Behaviours*. In Predicting Health

Behaviour. *Open University Press*, 2005. Bucking.

Coleman, L; Testa, A. Sexual health knowledge, attitudes and behaviours among an ethnically diverse sample of young people in the UK. *Health Education Journal*, 2007;66 (1): 68-81

Edelman, C.L. and Mandle, C.L. (2006). *Health promotion throughout the life span*. 6th ed. St. Louis: Mosby Inc.
Morrison,A; Macki,C.M; Elliot,L et al., The Sexual Health Centre: a service for young people. *Journal of Public Health*, 2006;19 (4): 457-463

Nester Murira obtained her PhD from Birmingham City University, UK. She has a Masters' Degree in Medical Education from Dundee University, Scotland, and a B.Ed.in Adult Education from University of Zimbabwe. Nester has worked in reproductive health as a clinician, a researcher and a lecturer. She has written several health promotion books for children, adolescents and adults as well as professional books for midwives. She also writes children's story books. Nester is also a copywriter.